CONTENTS

INTRODUCTION TO PSILOCYBIN MUSHROOMS

Understanding Psilocybin and Its Effects

Psilocybin, a naturally occurring psychedelic compound found in certain species of mushrooms, has garnered significant attention for its mind-altering properties. This compound interacts with serotonin receptors in the brain, leading to perceptual changes, altered thinking patterns, and profound spiritual experiences.

Psilocybin's Mechanism of Action

1. **Serotonin Receptor Agonism:** Psilocybin is metabolized into psilocin in the body, which acts as a partial agonist at serotonin receptors, particularly the 5-HT2A receptor. This activation induces alterations in neural activity, leading to changes in perception and mood.

2. **Neuroplasticity and Connectivity:** Studies suggest that psilocybin facilitates increased communication between brain regions that don't typically interact. This heightened connectivity may underlie the vivid hallucinations and novel thought patterns experienced during a trip.

3. **Psychological Effects:** Psilocybin ingestion can lead to various experiences, from euphoria and introspection to anxiety and paranoia. The impact is influenced by set (the user's mindset) and setting (the environment).

4. **Therapeutic Potential:** Recent research has explored psilocybin's therapeutic applications in treating conditions like depression, anxiety, PTSD, and addiction. Clinical trials have shown promising results in managing these mental health disorders.

Historical Significance and Cultural Context

The use of psilocybin-containing mushrooms dates back centuries and holds cultural and spiritual significance in various indigenous societies across the globe.

Traditional Use and Rituals

1. **Indigenous Practices:** Indigenous cultures in Central and South America, like the Aztecs and Maya, used psilocybin mushrooms ceremonially for religious rituals, healing, and divination purposes.

2. **Spiritual Significance:** Psilocybin mushrooms were revered for their perceived ability to facilitate communication with spiritual realms, inducing altered states of consciousness for

guidance and enlightenment.

3. **Western Discovery:** Psilocybin gained attention in the Western world during the mid-20th century when researchers and countercultural movements embraced it as a tool for expanding consciousness and exploring the mind.

4. **Psychedelic Renaissance:** In recent years, there's been a resurgence of interest in psychedelics, including psilocybin, for their potential therapeutic benefits, sparking a renewed exploration of ancient practices in modern clinical settings.

Legal Framework and Current Status

The legal status of psilocybin varies significantly across different jurisdictions, with some places considering it a controlled substance while others are exploring decriminalization or regulated use.

Global Legal Landscape

1. **Legal Status:** In most countries, psilocybin-containing mushrooms are classified as illegal substances, with severe penalties for possession, cultivation, or distribution.

2. **Decriminalization Efforts:** Certain cities and regions have pursued decriminalization initiatives, aiming to reduce penalties associated with possession and personal use while prioritizing education and harm reduction.

3. **Research and Medical Use:** Despite legal restrictions, some countries allow psilocybin

research for medical purposes under strict regulations. This leniency has enabled clinical trials and studies to explore its therapeutic potential.

4. **Changing Perspectives:** There's a growing movement advocating for policy changes, emphasizing the need for evidence-based approaches to reconsider the legal status of psilocybin, especially in the context of its potential medical benefits.

Understanding psilocybin and its effects encompasses scientific, cultural, and legal dimensions. As research continues and societal attitudes evolve, the discourse surrounding this compound is evolving, shedding light on its complexities and potential contributions to mental health treatment and human consciousness.

SCIENCE OF PSILOCYBIN MUSHROOMS

Chemical Composition and Neurological Impact

Understanding the chemical composition of substances and their neurological impact is crucial for comprehending how various compounds interact with the brain and nervous system. Chemicals, both naturally occurring and synthetic, can have profound effects on brain function and behavior. The human brain's intricate network of neurons and neurotransmitters forms the basis of neurological responses to these compounds.

Neurotransmitters and Brain Chemistry

Neurotransmitters play a pivotal role in transmitting

signals across the brain. **Dopamine, serotonin, and acetylcholine** are prominent neurotransmitters influencing mood, cognition, and behavior. The chemical composition of these neurotransmitters involves specific molecular structures that dictate their functions. For instance, dopamine contributes to motivation and reward pathways, serotonin regulates mood and emotions, while acetylcholine plays a role in memory and learning.

Understanding how the chemical composition of these neurotransmitters interacts with receptors in the brain is fundamental. **Receptors such as G-protein-coupled receptors and ionotropic receptors** respond differently to various compounds, influencing neurological responses. Chemicals can act as agonists or antagonists, mimicking or inhibiting neurotransmitter functions, respectively, altering brain activity and impacting neurological processes.

Synthetic Compounds and Neurological Effects

Synthetic compounds, such as pharmaceutical drugs or illicit substances, often mimic or interfere with natural neurotransmitters, affecting brain chemistry and neurological functions. **Opioids, amphetamines, and cannabinoids** are examples of synthetic compounds with diverse neurological impacts. Opioids interact with opioid receptors, modulating pain perception and inducing euphoria, but they also carry the risk of addiction and respiratory depression.

Amphetamines influence dopamine and norepinephrine levels, leading to increased alertness and euphoria, but prolonged use can result in tolerance and dependence. Cannabinoids, like THC (tetrahydrocannabinol), affect the endocannabinoid system, impacting mood, memory, and perception. These synthetic compounds demonstrate how alterations in brain chemistry can lead to both desired effects and adverse consequences.

Environmental Toxins and Neurological Health

Beyond intentional consumption, exposure to environmental toxins can also impact neurological health. **Heavy metals like lead and mercury**, pesticides, and air pollutants have been linked to neurological disorders. The chemical composition of these toxins allows them to infiltrate the nervous system, disrupting neuronal function and potentially leading to conditions such as developmental delays, cognitive impairments, and neurodegenerative diseases.

Understanding the chemical properties of these toxins and their mechanisms of action within the nervous system is crucial for preventing and mitigating their adverse neurological effects. Efforts to limit exposure and develop treatments to counteract their impact remain critical in safeguarding neurological health.

Therapeutic Potential: Medical and Psychological

Exploring the therapeutic potential of various compounds for medical and psychological purposes has been a focal point in scientific research. From pharmaceutical drugs to natural remedies, compounds have been investigated for their ability to alleviate symptoms, manage conditions, and promote well-being, both physically and mentally.

Medicinal Compounds and Treatment

Antidepressants, antipsychotics, and analgesics are examples of medicinal compounds used to address psychological and physical ailments. Antidepressants, such as SSRIs (selective serotonin reuptake inhibitors), modulate serotonin levels, aiding in managing depression and anxiety disorders. Antipsychotics target dopamine receptors, assisting in managing symptoms of schizophrenia and bipolar disorder.

Analgesics, including opioids and nonsteroidal anti-inflammatory drugs (NSAIDs), are employed to alleviate pain. Despite their effectiveness, the use of opioids for pain management has been accompanied by concerns regarding addiction and overdose, prompting exploration into alternative pain relief strategies.

Natural Remedies and Holistic Approaches

Natural remedies derived from plants and herbs have garnered attention for their potential therapeutic effects. **Herbal supplements like St. John's Wort for depression**, turmeric for its anti-inflammatory properties, and CBD (cannabidiol) for anxiety and pain relief have been subjects of research.

Holistic approaches encompass practices like acupuncture, meditation, and yoga, emphasizing the mind-body connection for overall well-being. These practices leverage the body's natural mechanisms, impacting neurotransmitter release, stress reduction, and promoting relaxation, thus potentially contributing to psychological and physical health.

Psychedelics and Mental Health Exploration

Research into psychedelics like psilocybin (found in certain mushrooms) and LSD (lysergic acid diethylamide) has gained traction for their potential in mental health therapy. These compounds, known for their hallucinogenic properties, have shown promise in **treating depression, PTSD, and substance use disorders**.

Their unique neurological impact involves altering perception and inducing introspection, potentially facilitating therapeutic breakthroughs. Studies suggest that these compounds may foster neuroplasticity, enabling new connections in the brain and prompting novel approaches to mental health treatment.

Studies and Research Findings

Advancements in technology and methodologies have facilitated extensive studies and research, providing insights into the complex interactions between compounds and neurological systems. Scientific investigations have elucidated various facets of chemical composition, neurological impacts, and therapeutic potentials, contributing to the understanding of brain function and disorders.

Neuroimaging Techniques and Insights

Neuroimaging techniques like **fMRI (functional magnetic resonance imaging)** and PET (positron emission tomography) scans have enabled researchers to visualize brain activity and chemical processes. These tools offer a window into how compounds influence neural pathways, revealing correlations between chemical interactions and observed neurological responses.

These studies have highlighted the brain regions involved in specific tasks, emotions, and disorders. For instance, observing increased dopamine release in reward pathways during pleasurable experiences or identifying aberrant activity in certain brain regions linked to psychiatric conditions has deepened our understanding of neurological function and dysfunction.

Clinical Trials and Efficacy Assessments

Clinical trials evaluating the efficacy and safety of compounds have been pivotal in shaping medical and psychological treatments. **Randomized controlled trials (RCTs)** and longitudinal studies assess the effects of compounds on patient populations, providing valuable data on both short-term and long-term impacts.

These studies aid in determining optimal dosage, identifying potential side effects, and assessing overall treatment efficacy. Research findings from such trials inform medical guidelines and contribute to evidence-based practices in healthcare, guiding clinicians in prescribing appropriate interventions for patients.

Meta-Analyses and Comprehensive Reviews

Meta-analyses and comprehensive reviews synthesize findings from multiple studies, offering a broader perspective on compound effects and neurological impacts. **Pooling data from various research endeavors** allows for a more comprehensive assessment of trends, potential biases, and inconsistencies within the literature.

These analyses aid in drawing more robust conclusions, identifying gaps in knowledge, and guiding future research directions. They serve as valuable resources for researchers, clinicians, and policymakers in making informed decisions regarding treatments, interventions, and regulations.

IDENTIFYING AND CLASSIFYING PSILOCYBIN MUSHROOMS

Species Overview and Differentiation of Psilocybin Mushrooms

Psilocybin mushrooms, commonly referred to as magic mushrooms or shrooms, belong to a group of fungi that contain psychoactive compounds. The most prevalent species known for their psilocybin content include Psilocybe cubensis, Psilocybe semilanceata (also known as liberty cap), and Psilocybe cyanescens. Each species possesses distinct characteristics that aid in identification.

Psilocybe cubensis is one of the most widespread and recognizable species. It typically features a bell-shaped cap with a distinct caramel or chestnut brown color. The cap can range from 1 to 8 centimeters in diameter and has a convex or flattened shape as it matures. The gills underneath the cap are initially whitish, progressing to a dark purplish-brown as the mushroom matures. Its stem is long and thick, often exhibiting a white or pale yellow hue.

Psilocybe semilanceata, commonly known as the liberty cap, is smaller in size compared to Psilocybe cubensis. Its cap is conical or bell-shaped, with a pointy tip, and ranges from 0.5 to 2 centimeters in diameter. The color of the cap varies from light brown to yellowish-green, and it often has a distinct nipple-like protrusion at the center. Its stem is slender and elongated, featuring a pale hue.

Psilocybe cyanescens is recognized for its wavy, undulating cap, ranging from 1 to 4 centimeters in diameter. The color of the cap varies from light brown to caramel or chestnut, with a distinct hygrophanous nature —changing color based on moisture levels. Its stem is thicker at the base and tapers towards the top, featuring a whitish or pale yellow coloration.

Distinguishing between these species is crucial due to variations in potency, growing conditions, and geographic prevalence. Utilizing expert resources and detailed identification guides is paramount for accurately differentiating between these mushrooms.

Habitat, Growth Conditions, and Ecology of Psilocybin Mushrooms

Psilocybin mushrooms thrive in diverse habitats across the globe, favoring specific environmental conditions for growth. They often grow in moist, humid environments such as forests, grasslands, and decaying organic matter like dung, wood chips, or compost. Understanding their growth conditions is vital for cultivation and recognizing their ecological significance.

Key factors influencing their growth include:

1. **Moisture:** Psilocybin mushrooms require high humidity levels to flourish. Adequate moisture content in the substrate or environment is essential for successful growth.

2. **Temperature:** Moderate temperatures between 15 to 30 degrees Celsius (59 to 86 degrees Fahrenheit) support optimal mushroom growth. Extreme temperatures can inhibit their development.

3. **Substrate:** Different species of psilocybin mushrooms have specific substrate preferences. For instance, Psilocybe cubensis often grows in nutrient-rich substrates like composted manure or decaying plant matter.

In terms of ecology, these mushrooms play a pivotal role in nutrient cycling and decomposition processes. They aid in breaking down organic matter, facilitating nutrient release and soil enrichment. Additionally, they form symbiotic relationships with certain plant species, contributing to the overall health and biodiversity of ecosystems.

Understanding the ecological niche and growth requirements of psilocybin mushrooms is vital for conservation efforts and responsible cultivation practices.

Visual Identification and Safety Measures of Psilocybin Mushrooms

Accurate visual identification is crucial when foraging

for psilocybin mushrooms due to the existence of both psychoactive and poisonous species. Developing a keen eye for recognizing distinguishing features while adhering to safety measures is imperative to avoid accidental ingestion of toxic varieties.

Key features for visual identification include:

1. **Cap Characteristics:** Examining the shape, size, and color of the cap is essential. Variations in color, texture, and shape can differentiate between species.

2. **Gill Structure:** The arrangement, color, and attachment of gills beneath the cap are important indicators.

3. **Stem Attributes:** Observing the stem's color, thickness, and any distinctive markings or remnants of a partial veil helps in identification.

4. **Bruising Reaction:** Psilocybin-containing mushrooms typically exhibit a bluing or bruising reaction when handled or damaged.

Safety measures to consider when identifying psilocybin mushrooms:

1. **Consult Experts:** Seek guidance from experienced mycologists or reliable identification resources before foraging or consuming any wild mushrooms.

2. **Use Field Guides:** Refer to comprehensive field guides with detailed descriptions and high-quality images for accurate identification.

3. **Start Small:** If one is new to mushroom foraging,

it's advisable to start by identifying well-known species and gradually expand knowledge.

4. **Avoid Assumptions:** Never consume mushrooms solely based on appearance or assumptions. Always double-check identification through multiple reliable sources

CULTIVATION AND PROPAGATION TECHNIQUES

Growing Psilocybin Mushrooms: Methods and Practices

Psilocybin mushrooms, known for their psychoactive properties, have gained attention for their potential therapeutic benefits. Growing these mushrooms involves several methods and practices that require precision, attention to detail, and a suitable environment.

Methods of Cultivation

1. Substrate Preparation:

Psilocybin mushrooms typically grow on substrates like grain, straw, or compost. Grains like rye or millet are popular choices. The substrate needs sterilization to eliminate competing organisms. It can be achieved through pressure cooking or boiling.

2. Inoculation and Colonization:

Once the substrate is prepared, it's inoculated with mushroom spores or mycelium culture. This step requires aseptic techniques to prevent contamination. The mycelium then colonizes the substrate, forming a network of threads.

3. Fruiting Conditions:

After colonization, providing proper fruiting conditions is crucial. Maintaining the right temperature, humidity, and light exposure stimulates mushroom growth. Mist chambers or grow tents are often used to control these factors.

4. Harvesting Techniques:

Harvesting should be done carefully, avoiding damage to the mycelium. Mushrooms are typically picked just before the veil underneath the cap breaks. This timing ensures peak potency.

Tools, Equipment, and Setup

1. Pressure Cooker or Autoclave:

Sterilization of substrates requires high temperatures to kill unwanted organisms. Pressure cookers or autoclaves are essential tools for ensuring sterile conditions.

2. Mason Jars or Bags:

These containers hold the substrate during the colonization process. They should be heat resistant and airtight to prevent contamination.

3. Grow Lights:

Proper lighting mimics natural conditions, aiding in the growth of psilocybin mushrooms. LED grow lights with adjustable settings for different growth stages are commonly used.

4. Hygrometer and Thermometer:

Monitoring humidity and temperature levels is crucial. Hygrometers and thermometers help maintain optimal conditions for mushroom growth.

5. Grow Tents or Chambers:

Controlling the environment is easier with grow tents or chambers. These structures help regulate humidity, temperature, and light exposure, creating an ideal setting for mushroom cultivation.

Harvesting, Preservation, and Storage Tips

1. Timing of Harvest:

Harvesting at the right time ensures maximum potency. The veil breaking beneath the cap indicates the ideal time for picking mushrooms.

2. Drying Techniques:

Proper drying prevents mold growth and preserves potency. Techniques include using a dehydrator, silica gel, or desiccant packs in a well-ventilated area.

3. Storage Containers:

Opt for airtight containers like glass jars to store dried mushrooms. Keep them away from moisture, light, and heat to maintain potency.

4. Rehydration Process:

When ready to use, rehydrate mushrooms by soaking them in water for a short period. This step can revive their texture and potency.

5. Long-term Preservation:

For long-term storage, consider vacuum-sealing dried mushrooms and storing them in a cool, dark place. This helps preserve their potency for an extended period.

In the realm of growing psilocybin mushrooms, these methods and practices form a foundation for successful cultivation. Precision and attention to detail at each stage, from substrate preparation to harvesting and storage, are imperative for obtaining high-quality yields with maximum potency.

CONSUMPTION AND DOSAGE GUIDELINES

*Various Methods of Ingesting
Psilocybin Mushrooms
and Their Effects*

Psilocybin mushrooms, commonly known as "magic mushrooms," have been used for centuries due to their psychoactive properties. The methods of ingestion vary, each influencing the onset, duration, and intensity of the experience.

1. Oral Ingestion:

The most traditional and straightforward method is oral consumption. **This can be done through:**

- **Eating Raw:** Chewing and swallowing the mushrooms in their natural state.
- **Brewing Tea:** Steeping the mushrooms in hot water to make a potent brew.

- **Mixing in Food:** Incorporating mushrooms into various dishes to mask the taste.

Effects: Oral ingestion typically takes 20-40 minutes to kick in, with effects lasting 4-6 hours. The intensity can vary based on dosage and individual tolerance. Users often report altered perception, euphoria, enhanced creativity, and spiritual experiences.

2. Smoking or Vaporizing:

Some individuals opt for unconventional methods such as smoking or vaporizing psilocybin mushrooms. **This involves:**

- **Drying and Smoking:** Drying mushrooms and smoking them in a joint or pipe.
- **Vaporization:** Using specialized devices to heat mushrooms without combustion, inhaling the vapors.

Effects: Smoking or vaporizing psilocybin mushrooms leads to a quicker onset, usually within minutes. The experience tends to be shorter, lasting 2-3 hours. Users report a rapid but intense psychedelic experience, often with a stronger peak.

3. Microdosing:

Microdosing involves taking small, sub-perceptual amounts of psilocybin regularly over an extended period.

This method entails:

- **Careful Dosage:** Ingesting minimal amounts, typically one-tenth to one-twentieth of a recreational dose.

- **Regular Schedule:** Taking the microdose every few days or following a specific schedule.

Effects: Microdosing aims to enhance creativity, focus, and mood while avoiding strong psychoactive effects. Users often report improved cognition, increased energy, and emotional balance without significant impairment in daily functioning.

Dosage Calculations and Administration

Determining the appropriate dosage is crucial to achieve the desired effects while minimizing risks. Psilocybin potency can vary between species and individual mushrooms. **Dosage considerations include:**

- **Start Low:** Begin with a small dose, gradually increasing if needed.
- **Consider Tolerance:** Individual tolerance levels may vary due to factors like body weight and metabolism.
- **Psilocybin Content:** Different species and strains contain varying concentrations of psilocybin, influencing dosage.
- **Set and Setting:** The environment and mental state can affect the overall experience, requiring adjustments in dosage.

Administration Methods: Dosages are measured in grams of dried mushrooms or micrograms of pure psilocybin. Precise measurement and accuracy are crucial to avoid accidental ingestion of excessive amounts.

Safety Measures and Risk Mitigation

While psilocybin mushrooms are considered relatively safe compared to many other substances, there are still risks associated with their use. Employing safety measures is vital to minimize potential adverse effects.

1. Set and Setting:

- **Mindset:** Ensuring a positive and stable mental state before ingestion.
- **Setting:** Choosing a comfortable and safe environment, preferably with trusted company.

2. Trip Sitting:

- **Having a Guide:** Designating a sober and experienced individual to assist during the experience.
- **Support:** Providing reassurance and assistance if needed, especially for first-time users.

3. Personal Health Considerations:

- **Pre-existing Conditions:** Individuals with mental health issues or certain medical conditions should use caution or avoid psilocybin use altogether.
- **Medication Interactions:** Being aware of potential interactions with medications is crucial to prevent adverse reactions.

4. Integration and Aftercare:

- **Integration:** Reflecting on the experience and integrating insights gained into daily life.
- **Self-Care:** Prioritizing rest, nutrition, and mental well-being after the experience.

SPIRITUAL AND CULTURAL IMPLICATIONS

Psilocybin Mushrooms in Traditional and Modern Practices

Psilocybin mushrooms, also known as magic mushrooms, have a rich history deeply entwined with traditional practices across various cultures worldwide. These fungi contain psychoactive compounds like psilocybin and psilocin, known to induce altered states of consciousness. In traditional settings, these mushrooms were revered for their spiritual and healing properties. The traditional use of psilocybin mushrooms spans ancient civilizations such as the Aztecs in Mesoamerica, where they were employed in religious ceremonies to connect with deities and gain spiritual insight. Similarly, indigenous tribes in Central and South America considered these mushrooms as sacred entities, facilitating communion with nature and enhancing tribal rituals. The reverence for psilocybin mushrooms in these cultures reflects a profound understanding of their potential for spiritual enlightenment and therapeutic purposes.

In modern times, the resurgence of interest in psychedelics has led to renewed exploration of psilocybin mushrooms' therapeutic potential. **Modern research and clinical studies** have focused on their use in treating mental health conditions like depression, anxiety, and PTSD. Controlled environments with trained therapists have shown promising results in leveraging the psychotherapeutic effects of psilocybin, aiding individuals in addressing deep-seated emotional issues and fostering personal growth. The integration of these mushrooms into modern psychotherapy has sparked discussions around their legalization and regulated use for therapeutic purposes, emphasizing their potential to revolutionize mental healthcare.

Personal Growth, Spirituality, and Psychedelic Experiences

The ingestion of psilocybin mushrooms often catalyzes profound and introspective experiences that contribute to personal growth and spiritual exploration. **Key elements of personal growth** facilitated by these experiences include heightened self-awareness, emotional release, and a sense of interconnectedness with the universe. Psychedelic trips are often characterized by ego dissolution, allowing individuals to transcend their sense of self and perceive reality from an expanded perspective. These experiences can lead to transformative insights, fostering empathy, and compassion towards oneself and others.

Spirituality and psychedelic experiences share a

close relationship, as many individuals report mystical encounters and transcendent moments while under the influence of psilocybin mushrooms. The dissolution of boundaries between the self and the cosmos can evoke spiritual revelations, leading to a deeper understanding of existential questions and one's place in the universe. These experiences have been likened to religious or mystical awakenings, guiding individuals towards spiritual growth and a renewed sense of purpose.

Societal Impact and Contemporary Relevance

The societal impact of psilocybin mushrooms has sparked discussions on their contemporary relevance and potential implications for culture, policy, and public health. **Contemporary societal attitudes** towards psychedelics have evolved, shifting from stigma and criminalization towards a more nuanced understanding of their therapeutic value. Advocates and researchers have emphasized the need for responsible and regulated access to these substances, highlighting their potential to address the growing mental health crisis.

Legal and policy considerations surrounding the use of psilocybin mushrooms vary across different regions. Some jurisdictions have initiated measures to decriminalize or legalize these substances for therapeutic or research purposes, while others maintain stringent prohibitions. The ongoing discourse on the societal impact involves balancing public health concerns, individual rights, and scientific advancements in understanding the therapeutic potential of these mushrooms

PSILOCYBIN AND MENTAL HEALTH APPLICATIONS

Psilocybin, a naturally occurring psychedelic compound found in certain species of mushrooms, has gained attention in recent years for its potential therapeutic effects. Psilocybin-assisted therapy involves the use of this compound in a controlled setting to treat various mental health conditions. The methods employed in this therapy typically include careful dosing, psychological preparation, and structured guidance throughout the experience.

Dosage Protocols: One key aspect of psilocybin-assisted therapy is establishing proper dosage protocols. Research suggests that the dosage significantly impacts the therapeutic outcomes. Studies often administer a moderate to high dose of psilocybin, usually between 20 to

30 milligrams per 70 kilograms of body weight, to induce the desired effects without overwhelming the participant. The timing and frequency of dosing sessions are also vital considerations, with intervals between sessions allowing for integration and processing.

Set and Setting: The psychological state of the individual (set) and the environment (setting) play crucial roles in the efficacy of psilocybin-assisted therapy. Patients undergo thorough psychological preparation to cultivate a positive mindset and intention before the session. The setting is carefully designed to be comfortable, safe, and conducive to introspection, often including soothing music, dim lighting, and the presence of trained therapists to provide support and guidance throughout the experience.

Therapeutic Mechanisms: Psilocybin interacts with serotonin receptors in the brain, particularly the 5-HT2A receptor, leading to alterations in consciousness and perception. This neurobiological effect is believed to facilitate profound introspection, emotional release, and enhanced cognitive flexibility during the therapeutic session. The altered state of consciousness experienced under the influence of psilocybin allows individuals to explore deep-seated thoughts and emotions, potentially leading to insights and psychological breakthroughs.

Clinical Results and Efficacy: Numerous studies have shown promising results in using psilocybin-assisted therapy for various mental health conditions, including treatment-resistant depression, anxiety disorders, PTSD, and addiction. Clinical trials have reported significant improvements in mood, reduction in symptoms, and increased overall well-being in participants. For instance, trials conducted at reputable institutions have demonstrated rapid and sustained antidepressant effects in patients with major depressive disorder following psilocybin-assisted therapy.

Case Studies, Success Stories, and Clinical Trials

Case Studies: Individual case studies provide anecdotal evidence of the potential benefits of psilocybin-assisted therapy. These stories often highlight personal transformations, profound insights, and long-lasting positive changes in individuals struggling with mental health issues. For example, documented cases showcase how individuals experiencing severe depression or existential distress found relief and renewed perspectives after undergoing psilocybin-assisted therapy.

Success Stories: Success stories from participants who have undergone psilocybin-assisted therapy often emphasize the transformative nature of the experience. These narratives frequently describe a sense of profound connectedness, resolution of past traumas, and a newfound appreciation for life. Success stories contribute to the growing body of qualitative evidence supporting the therapeutic potential of psilocybin.

Clinical Trials: Rigorous clinical trials conducted in controlled settings offer empirical evidence regarding the safety and efficacy of psilocybin-assisted therapy. These trials follow strict methodologies, including randomized control groups, placebo administration, and long-term follow-ups to assess the sustained effects of the therapy. Several well-designed trials have shown statistically significant improvements in mental health outcomes among participants compared to control groups.

Future Prospects in Mental Health Treatment

Integration into Mainstream Healthcare: The future of psilocybin-assisted therapy in mental health treatment looks promising, with increasing interest from researchers, clinicians, and regulatory bodies. Efforts are underway to integrate this therapy into mainstream healthcare, albeit with necessary regulatory frameworks and standardized protocols to ensure safety and efficacy.

Advancements in Research: Ongoing research continues to explore the mechanisms of action of psilocybin and its potential applications in treating a wider range of mental health conditions. This includes investigating optimal dosing regimens, identifying patient populations most likely to benefit, and exploring the long-term effects of psilocybin-assisted therapy on mental health outcomes.

Public Perception and Education: Addressing stigma and misconceptions surrounding psychedelics remains a challenge. Education and public awareness campaigns are crucial to inform the general populace and healthcare professionals about the science behind psilocybin-assisted therapy. Increased understanding and acceptance may pave the way for wider adoption and accessibility of this treatment modality.

Collaboration and Regulation: Collaboration between researchers, healthcare providers, regulatory agencies, and pharmaceutical companies is essential to navigate the legal and ethical complexities associated with the therapeutic use of psilocybin. Striking a balance between innovation and safety through appropriate regulation will be pivotal in shaping the future landscape of mental health treatment.

POTENTIAL RISKS AND PRECAUTIONS

*Addressing Common
Misconceptions and Myths
about Psilocybin Mushrooms*

Psilocybin mushrooms, also known as magic mushrooms, have a long-standing association with myths and misconceptions. One common misconception is that they are highly addictive. However, research indicates that psilocybin itself isn't addictive. Unlike substances such as nicotine or opioids, psilocybin doesn't create compulsive drug-seeking behavior in users. It's crucial to distinguish between addiction and psychological dependence. While individuals might seek repeated experiences due to the psychological effects, it's not addiction in the traditional sense.

Another prevalent myth surrounds the dangers of psilocybin mushrooms, claiming that they are inherently lethal. **In reality, fatal overdoses from psilocybin mushrooms are extremely rare.** The LD50 (lethal dose for

50% of the population) of psilocybin is considerably high compared to many other substances. The risks of fatality primarily come from accidents or risky behavior during the altered state induced by the mushrooms rather than from the compound itself.

One misconception often propagated is that psilocybin mushrooms lead to permanent mental health issues, such as triggering psychosis or schizophrenia. **Current research does not support this claim.** While there's evidence suggesting that individuals with a predisposition to certain mental health conditions might experience exacerbation of symptoms, it's not considered a direct cause. However, caution is necessary for individuals with a personal or family history of psychotic disorders when using psychedelics.

A common misunderstanding revolves around the legality of psilocybin mushrooms. **Many assume that psilocybin mushrooms are entirely illegal everywhere.** However, there are regions and countries where certain forms or amounts might be decriminalized or legal for medical or religious purposes. It's crucial to understand the legal status in a specific area before assuming their legality or illegality.

Health Risks and Adverse Effects

Understanding the potential health risks and adverse effects associated with psilocybin mushrooms is crucial for responsible use. **The most commonly reported adverse effects include nausea, increased heart rate, and anxiety during the experience.** However, these effects are typically short-lived and tend to diminish as the psychedelic effects subside.

Another point to consider is the potential for a "bad trip." This refers to a distressing or overwhelming psychedelic experience. Factors such as set (mindset), setting (environment), and dosage play crucial roles in determining the nature of the trip. While challenging, a bad trip is not necessarily harmful in the long term, and providing a safe, supportive environment can help manage and mitigate its effects.

There's ongoing debate about the impact of psilocybin on mental health, particularly regarding its potential to alleviate or exacerbate existing conditions. **While some studies suggest therapeutic benefits for conditions like depression, anxiety, and PTSD, there are concerns about triggering latent mental health issues in susceptible individuals.** It's essential to approach the use of psilocybin mushrooms cautiously, especially for those with pre-existing mental health conditions.

Additionally, interaction with other medications or substances is a significant consideration. Psilocybin can interact with certain medications, including antidepressants and other psychotropic drugs, leading to adverse effects or reduced efficacy. Consultation with a healthcare professional is advisable before combining psilocybin mushrooms with any medication.

Risk Management Strategies

Mitigating risks associated with psilocybin mushroom use involves implementing various strategies:

Education and Preparation: Providing comprehensive information about the effects, potential risks, and harm reduction strategies is crucial. Education empowers individuals to make informed decisions and prepare for their experiences.

Dosage and Setting: Encouraging responsible dosing and emphasizing the importance of a safe, comfortable setting can significantly influence the overall experience. A controlled environment with trusted individuals reduces the likelihood of negative outcomes.

Screening and Support: Prioritizing the well-being of individuals by screening for underlying mental health conditions and providing adequate support and guidance during and after the experience can contribute to risk reduction.

Integration and Follow-up: Offering integration sessions after the psychedelic experience allows individuals to process and integrate insights gained during the trip, minimizing potential adverse effects and maximizing the therapeutic benefits.

Legal Awareness: Understanding and adhering to local laws and regulations regarding psilocybin mushrooms is essential to avoid legal repercussions and ensure responsible use within permissible boundaries.

ETHICAL AND LEGAL CONSIDERATIONS

Legal Frameworks and Regulations Worldwide on Psilocybin Mushrooms

Psilocybin mushrooms, commonly known as magic mushrooms, have gained attention due to their potential therapeutic benefits. However, the legal status of psilocybin varies significantly worldwide. Understanding the legal frameworks and regulations is crucial in navigating the complexities surrounding their use, possession, and distribution.

Regulatory Landscape

1. Global Variances:

The legal stance on psilocybin mushrooms varies widely

across countries. Some nations, like the Netherlands and Portugal, have decriminalized or partially legalized their use, while others, like the United States and many Asian countries, classify them as controlled substances.

2. Decriminalization vs. Legalization:

Several jurisdictions have opted for decriminalization rather than outright legalization. This approach focuses on reducing penalties for possession while keeping distribution and sale illegal.

3. Medical and Research Exceptions:

Certain countries allow psilocybin for medical or research purposes under strict regulations. Institutions and researchers often need specific licenses and permissions to handle these substances.

4. Ongoing Legislative Changes:

Recent years have seen shifts in attitudes towards psychedelics, with some regions considering policy changes to allow therapeutic use or scientific research, reflecting a potential reevaluation of psilocybin's legal status.

Challenges and Controversies

1. Public Perception and Stigma:

One of the primary challenges stems from societal stigmas surrounding psychedelics. Misconceptions and historical prejudices have contributed to resistance against legalizing or decriminalizing psilocybin.

2. Law Enforcement and Implementation Issues:

Discrepancies between state and federal laws in some countries create confusion and challenges in enforcement.

Law enforcement faces difficulties in differentiating personal use from distribution or production activities.

3. Safety and Risk Concerns:

Regulators and policymakers grapple with assessing the safety and potential risks associated with psilocybin use. Balancing the therapeutic benefits against potential adverse effects poses a significant challenge.

4. International Collaboration and Harmonization:

Given the global nature of drug policies, achieving international collaboration and uniformity in regulating psilocybin remains a challenge. Harmonizing laws across nations could streamline research and access while ensuring public safety.

Ethical Dilemmas and Debates

The exploration of psilocybin's therapeutic potential raises various ethical questions and prompts debates on multiple fronts.

Moral and Ethical Considerations

1. Autonomy vs. Paternalism:

Discussions often revolve around the balance between individual autonomy and paternalistic intervention. Should individuals have the freedom to explore psilocybin therapy, or should regulations prioritize protecting them from potential risks?

2. Informed Consent and Vulnerable Populations:

Ethical concerns emerge regarding informed consent, especially concerning vulnerable groups like minors or individuals with mental health conditions. Ensuring adequate information and safeguarding those who might be more susceptible to adverse effects is critical.

3. Cultural and Indigenous Perspectives:

Psilocybin mushrooms hold cultural significance in various indigenous traditions. Ethical considerations encompass respecting and integrating these cultural perspectives into regulatory frameworks without exploitation or appropriation.

4. Equitable Access and Social Justice:

Debates also revolve around ensuring equitable access to psilocybin therapy. There are concerns about affordability and accessibility, particularly for marginalized communities.

Future Outlook and Policy Recommendations

Emerging Trends and Potential Shifts

1. Advancements in Research and Clinical Trials:

The growing body of scientific evidence supporting the therapeutic potential of psilocybin is likely to influence policy changes. Continued research and clinical trials may prompt regulators to reconsider their stance.

2. Public Opinion and Advocacy Efforts:

Changing societal attitudes and increased advocacy for psychedelic-assisted therapies could exert pressure on policymakers to reassess regulations. Public support might drive legislative reforms.

Policy Recommendations

1. Evidence-based Regulations:

Policies should be informed by rigorous scientific evidence to strike a balance between promoting therapeutic access and mitigating risks associated with psilocybin use.

2. Education and Harm Reduction Programs:

Implementing educational initiatives and harm reduction strategies could help mitigate potential risks associated with psilocybin use, ensuring informed decisions and safer practices.

3. Collaborative International Efforts:

Encouraging global cooperation among nations and regulatory bodies can facilitate consistent policies and standards, fostering responsible use and research practices.

4. Inclusive Stakeholder Engagement:

Policymakers should engage diverse stakeholders, including healthcare professionals, researchers, affected communities, and advocacy groups, in formulating comprehensive and inclusive regulations.

The evolving legal, ethical, and policy landscapes surrounding psilocybin mushrooms demand a delicate balance between facilitating therapeutic innovation and ensuring public safety and ethical considerations. As research progresses and societal perspectives evolve, navigating these multifaceted issues will be crucial in shaping future frameworks and regulations worldwide.

INTEGRATION AND POST-PSILOCYBIN EXPERIENCE

1. Connection with Nature: Many individuals report a heightened appreciation for nature post-psychedelic experience. Integrating this connection into daily life could involve spending more time outdoors, gardening, or simply being present in natural surroundings.

2. Mindfulness Practices: Practices like meditation, yoga, or breathwork can help individuals stay grounded and maintain a sense of presence, integrating the heightened awareness experienced during the psychedelic journey into their daily routine.

3. Creative Expression: Art, music, dance, or other forms of creative expression often become more profound post-psychedelic experiences. Integrating these outlets into daily life can facilitate ongoing emotional expression and personal exploration.

4. Altered Perspectives: The altered perceptions and expanded consciousness experienced during a trip can lead to shifts in perspective. Integrating these perspectives involves recognizing and adapting to new ways of thinking or viewing the world around us.

5. Meaningful Relationships: Psychedelic experiences can deepen connections with others. Integrating this into daily life might involve fostering more authentic, open, and meaningful relationships with friends, family, or the community.

Support Networks and Community Engagement

1. Psychedelic Integration Circles: These are groups specifically designed to support individuals in integrating psychedelic experiences. These circles offer a safe and non-judgmental environment to share experiences and insights.

2. Online Communities: The digital space hosts various online forums, social media groups, and platforms dedicated to psychedelic integration. These spaces offer a sense of community and shared experiences for individuals seeking guidance or connection.

3. Therapeutic Guidance: Seeking professional therapeutic guidance from counselors, therapists, or integration coaches who specialize in psychedelic experiences can offer personalized support and aid in navigating the complexities of integration.

4. Peer Support Groups: Local or virtual peer support groups consisting of individuals who have undergone similar experiences can provide invaluable support, validation, and shared wisdom in integrating psychedelic journeys.

5. Community Engagement: Actively engaging in communities that support psychedelic advocacy, harm reduction, or education can provide a sense of belonging and purpose, fostering a collective effort toward destigmatization and responsible use.

Continuing Personal Growth and Well-being

1. Self-Care Practices: Implementing self-care routines involving healthy habits, nutrition, exercise, and adequate sleep contributes to overall well-being and supports continued personal growth.

2. Lifelong Learning: Embracing a mindset of continuous learning and self-improvement fuels personal growth. This could involve reading, attending workshops, or pursuing educational opportunities that align with individual interests.

3. Emotional Intelligence: Enhancing emotional intelligence through practices like mindfulness, therapy, or self-reflection aids in understanding oneself better and fosters healthier relationships with others.

4. Integration of Insights: Actively applying the insights gained from psychedelic experiences into daily life fosters continued growth. Regularly revisiting and integrating these lessons helps in evolving one's perspectives and behavior.

5. Contribution and Service: Engaging in acts of service or contributing to causes larger than oneself can bring a sense of purpose and fulfillment, supporting ongoing personal growth and well-being.

In conclusion, the integration of psychedelic experiences into daily life is a multifaceted journey that involves reflection, behavioral changes, support networks, and continued personal growth. It's a process that requires patience, self-compassion, and an ongoing commitment to holistic well-being.

FAQ AND EXPERT INSIGHTS

Frequently Asked Questions
about Psilocybin Mushrooms

Psilocybin mushrooms, also known as magic mushrooms or shrooms, have garnered attention for their potential therapeutic and recreational use. As interest grows, so do the inquiries and concerns surrounding their effects, legality, and safety. Below, I'll address common questions, provide expert insights, and offer clarity on this intriguing subject.

1. What are Psilocybin Mushrooms?

Psilocybin mushrooms are a type of fungi containing psychoactive compounds like psilocybin and psilocin. They belong to various species, with the most well-known being Psilocybe cubensis and Psilocybe semilanceata. These mushrooms have been used for centuries in spiritual and religious ceremonies due to their hallucinogenic properties.

Psilocybin, once ingested, converts into psilocin in the

body, leading to altered perceptions, mood changes, and sometimes mystical or profound experiences. These effects are largely subjective and can vary widely based on dosage, set, and setting.

2. What are the Effects of Psilocybin Mushrooms?

The effects of psilocybin mushrooms can vary significantly from person to person. Common experiences include visual distortions, changes in perception of time, enhanced emotions, and altered thought patterns. Users might also encounter feelings of interconnectedness, euphoria, or spiritual awakening. However, adverse effects such as anxiety, paranoia, or nausea can occur, especially with higher doses or in susceptible individuals.

3. Are Psilocybin Mushrooms Legal?

Legality concerning psilocybin mushrooms differs across countries and regions. In many places, including the United States, they are classified as illegal substances due to their hallucinogenic properties and potential for abuse. However, some jurisdictions are reconsidering their stance, exploring decriminalization or legalization for medical or research purposes.

4. Can Psilocybin Mushrooms be Used for Therapeutic Purposes?

Research suggests that psilocybin mushrooms may have therapeutic potential for various mental health conditions like depression, anxiety, PTSD, and addiction. Studies have shown promising results in controlled settings, where guided therapy sessions accompany the ingestion of psilocybin. The psychedelic experience, when facilitated by trained professionals, could aid in introspection, emotional healing, and personal growth.

5. What Precautions Should be Taken When Using Psilocybin Mushrooms?

When consuming psilocybin mushrooms, several precautions should be considered for safety and a positive experience:

- **Dosage:** Start with a low dose to gauge sensitivity and effects. Gradually increase if necessary but avoid high doses initially.

- **Set and Setting:** The environment and mindset significantly influence the trip. Choose a comfortable, familiar, and safe space with trusted individuals.

- **Mental State:** Individuals with a history of mental health issues should approach psychedelics cautiously and ideally under professional supervision.

- **Integration:** After the experience, reflection and integration of insights into daily life are crucial for long-term benefits.

6. What Are the Risks Associated with Psilocybin Mushrooms?

While psilocybin mushrooms are generally considered safe when used responsibly, there are potential risks:

- **Bad Trips:** Unpleasant experiences can occur, leading to anxiety, paranoia, or confusion.

- **Physical Effects:** Nausea, increased heart rate, and potential allergic reactions are possible.

- **Psychological Impact:** Individuals predisposed to certain mental health conditions might experience exacerbation of symptoms.

7. Can Psilocybin Mushrooms be Addictive?

Unlike substances like opioids or nicotine, psilocybin

mushrooms are not considered physically addictive. However, psychological dependence can develop in some individuals who misuse or excessively rely on them for escape or coping mechanisms.

8. What is the Current Status of Psilocybin Research?

Recent years have seen a resurgence in scientific interest in psilocybin. Numerous studies have explored its potential therapeutic applications, neuroscience of psychedelic experiences, and their impact on mental health. Organizations and researchers are advocating for expanded access to further investigate its benefits and risks.

9. How Can Psilocybin be Administered?

Psilocybin mushrooms can be consumed raw, dried, or brewed into a tea. Precise dosing can be challenging due to variability in mushroom potency. Efforts are underway to develop standardized doses and alternative delivery methods, like capsules or microdosing regimens.

10. What are the Ethical Considerations Surrounding Psilocybin Use?

Ethical discussions revolve around access, safety, informed consent, and cultural sensitivity. Balancing individual freedoms with public health concerns, ensuring equitable access to potential therapies, and respecting indigenous cultural traditions are vital aspects being debated.

CONCLUSION AND LOOKING AHEAD

Summary of Key Takeaways on Psilocybin Mushrooms

Psilocybin mushrooms, commonly known as magic mushrooms, have garnered substantial attention in recent years due to their potential therapeutic and recreational use. Understanding the key takeaways from research and cultural shifts surrounding these fungi is imperative for a nuanced perspective.

Key Takeaways:

1. **Psychedelic Properties:**

Psilocybin mushrooms contain the psychoactive compound psilocybin, inducing alterations in perception, mood, and cognition. These effects vary widely among individuals, influenced by dosage, setting, and personal predispositions. Studies reveal its potential in treating mental health disorders, including depression, anxiety, and PTSD.

2. **Historical and Cultural Significance:**

Cultures worldwide have long used psilocybin mushrooms in spiritual, religious, and healing ceremonies. Indigenous communities in Central and South America integrated these fungi for centuries, recognizing their profound impact on consciousness and spiritual awakening.

3. **Legal and Medical Landscape:**

Legal perspectives on psilocybin are evolving. Some regions and countries have decriminalized or approved its therapeutic use under controlled settings. Research institutions and pharmaceutical companies are exploring psilocybin's therapeutic potential, initiating clinical trials for various mental health conditions.

4. **Safety and Potential Risks:**

Psilocybin is generally considered safe when consumed responsibly in controlled environments. However, adverse reactions can occur, such as anxiety, paranoia, or temporary confusion. Proper dosage, psychological preparedness, and a supportive environment are crucial to mitigate potential risks.

5. **Psychedelic Renaissance:**

The resurgence of interest in psychedelics signals a shift in societal attitudes toward mental health treatment. Advocacy groups, scientists, and policymakers are advocating for further research, emphasizing the therapeutic benefits of psilocybin and challenging stigmas surrounding psychedelic substances.

Explanations:

1. **Psychedelic Properties:**

Psilocybin, the active ingredient in magic mushrooms,

interacts with serotonin receptors in the brain, leading to altered perception, mood elevation, and changes in consciousness. Its therapeutic potential lies in its ability to promote neuroplasticity and facilitate emotional processing, potentially aiding in therapy for various mental health disorders.

2. **Historical and Cultural Significance:**

Indigenous cultures in Mesoamerica, such as the Aztecs and Mayans, considered psilocybin mushrooms sacred and utilized them in religious ceremonies for spiritual insight and healing. Understanding these cultural contexts provides valuable insights into the traditional use and reverence for these fungi.

3. **Legal and Medical Landscape:**

Recent studies demonstrating promising results in treating conditions like depression have sparked reconsideration of psilocybin's legal status. Several regions have initiated decriminalization measures or authorized supervised therapeutic use, acknowledging its potential as a breakthrough treatment modality.

4. **Safety and Potential Risks:**

While psilocybin is not considered addictive and has a low toxicity profile, its effects can be unpredictable. Set and setting, the user's mindset and the environment in which they consume the substance, greatly influence the experience. Responsible use under professional guidance minimizes adverse effects.

5. **Psychedelic Renaissance:**

The growing acceptance of psychedelics in therapeutic settings is reshaping mental health care paradigms.

Research institutions and investors are increasingly funding studies on psilocybin, fostering a new wave of scientific exploration into its therapeutic applications, potentially revolutionizing mental health treatment.

Future Trends and Developments

The landscape surrounding psilocybin mushrooms is continually evolving, with several emerging trends and potential future developments reshaping societal perceptions and scientific endeavors.

Anticipated Trends:

1. Expanded Research:

Expect an upsurge in scientific studies investigating psilocybin's mechanisms of action, therapeutic potential, and optimal dosing protocols. Research institutions, universities, and private entities will likely invest more resources into understanding its impact on mental health.

2. Mainstream Integration:

Increased public awareness and shifting attitudes toward mental health treatments may lead to more widespread acceptance of psilocybin-assisted therapy. This could prompt mainstream integration, with clinics offering supervised sessions and personalized treatment plans.

3. Legislative Changes:

Anticipate ongoing discussions and potential legislative changes surrounding the decriminalization or legalization of psilocybin for therapeutic purposes in various regions. Policy shifts may occur as more evidence supports its efficacy and safety.

4. Commercialization and Industry Growth:

As research progresses and legal barriers potentially ease, the pharmaceutical and wellness industries may witness a surge in products derived from psilocybin. This could range from pharmaceutical formulations to wellness retreats offering psychedelic-assisted therapies.

Future Developments:

1. Advanced Treatment Modalities:

Innovations in delivery mechanisms, such as microdosing protocols, personalized therapy, and controlled-release formulations, may enhance the therapeutic effectiveness of psilocybin while minimizing potential side effects.

2. Integration with Conventional Medicine:

Collaborations between psychedelic-assisted therapy and conventional psychiatric treatments could emerge, leading to integrated approaches that combine the benefits of psilocybin with established therapeutic modalities.

3. Continued Public Discourse:

Expect ongoing discussions and advocacy efforts emphasizing the importance of destigmatizing psychedelics, promoting education, and ensuring equitable access to psilocybin-assisted therapies.

4. Ethical and Regulatory Considerations:

As interest grows, ethical considerations regarding access, equity, and responsible use will necessitate robust regulatory frameworks to ensure safe and equitable access while preventing misuse and exploitation.

Final Thoughts and Encouragement

In conclusion, the discourse surrounding psilocybin mushrooms is multifaceted and evolving, encompassing scientific, cultural, and societal dimensions. As research progresses and attitudes shift, it's essential to maintain a balanced perspective that acknowledges both the potential therapeutic benefits and associated risks of these substances.

Encouraging responsible exploration and continued research while advocating for safe and regulated access to psilocybin-assisted therapies is crucial. Embracing a nuanced understanding, supported by robust scientific inquiry and cultural sensitivity, can pave the way for innovative mental health treatments while respecting the historical significance and diverse cultural perspectives surrounding these mushrooms.

Let's foster an environment that encourages dialogue, education, and responsible integration of psilocybin into mental health care, ensuring its potential benefits are accessible to those who may benefit while safeguarding against potential risks